GOD'S HANDCRAFTED JEWEL

Faith in the Face of Illness

Cathy Jewel Chatman

Table of Content

Acknowledgments

I would like to acknowledge my family and friends who helped me through the process of publishing my first book and supported me during my darkest hours of illness.

I love my family. They are an excellent source of encouragement and inspiration to me. My three girls Tiffany, Victoria, and Danielle – you fill my life with joy, smiles, and laughter. My granddaughter Aria Michelle, the center of my joy. My husband, Victor – you have been committed for over thirty years. I thank God for how we have reared our girls to love God and love their family.

To the rest of my family, my mother Minnie, my aunts and uncles resting in heaven, cousins, and family through marriage, I want to say thank you for your support. I love you all so very much.

I would like to thank the Vision Plan Institute. My God sent Sister in Christ Wilma J. Williams for partnering with me through this long-awaited process of publishing my first book.

I am blessed with so many amazing friends who are more like family to me. You all have supported me during my crisis and recovery period. Thank you all so very much!

Introduction

Genesis 6:3 confirms that we can live to be 120 years old if we chose. This Word revelation has granted me a new birth date, April 24, 2008. On this day God blessed me to reclaim my longevity. I am a Stage 4 Breast Cancer Survivor. In the face of this terminal illness diagnosis, I experienced how God rules and reigns over our lives through His supernatural power. He proved himself to be Jehovah-Rapha, *My Healer.* God's supernatural healing power manifested in my life, and as my faith grew, I embraced my wellness more and more.

During my devotional time with God in 2008, God downloaded thoughts, affirmations, and scriptures that breathed life back into my weary soul. I pray you will experience revelation while reading my testimony. I pray you will be encouraged to embrace wellness and reclaim your life's longevity through faith. Fear not and know God is with you. He has plans for your life in the face of your diagnosis or any other crisis in your life.

I encourage you to not only protect your eye and ear gates but be mindful of the words that come out of your mouth. Your words, positive or negative, have power in them and affect the lives of everyone who hears them, including you. Walking in faith and standing firm on the Word of God in the face of illness was not easy. There were many days I had to block out everything around me to hear what God was saying through the Holy Spirit.

To stand in victory, in the midst of crisis, I decided to allow God's life-sustaining scriptures to be my weapon. I used God's handcrafted affirmations, such as Psalm 91:16 (With long life will God satisfy me and show me His great salvation) and Exodus 23:24-25 (I am blessed, and the Lord has taken sickness away from me), to declare victory over my life daily. I wrote them in a daily journal. I took on the mind of Christ.

CHAPTER 1

Life's Mortality

I could not believe this was happening to me, Cathy Jewel Chatman. After years confessing the Word of God, trusting and believing Him for financial security, it had come to pass. I felt secure in the blessings He had bestowed upon my life. The desires of my heart for my career had manifested. I received three promotions within the first thirty-days of working for s chain hair salon as a professional cosmetologist. One promotion afforded me to be the General Manager of three stores. This was the first time, since meeting my husband, I felt validated through my career accomplishment. I believe God was rewarding me for putting my career on hold, rearing my children up in the adoration of Christ, and being submissive to my husband. I felt good about the virtuous woman I had become.

I had been a homemaker for many years, my confidence as a woman, wife, mother, and daughter was through the roof. I was in the best physical shape I could be in. I was enjoying my life of healthy eating, holistic supplements, and spiritual growth. I was a major financial contributor in my household. The poverty I experienced as a child would never be my daughter's portion! My husband and I were at a point in our lives when money was not an

3

issue, and we could afford anything that we desired. My career was finally taking off, I was in a new position in my career and life was good. My husband and I were on our way to making decisions for our lives which included plans for our dream home and blessing our family and friends who are like family. Then the unexpected happened. The reality of my life's mortality was staring me in the face in the form of a lump in my breast. I could not wrap my mind around the possibility of an adverse diagnosis without imagining all the plans that would be lost. I never expected my life to be changed so drastically by a health diagnosis.

On December 31, 2007, I came home from work extremely tired. Work had been a sprint all day and the time flew by in a frantic blur. I miss interpreted the number of Clients needing a haircut preparing for New Year's Eve festivities that day. We were not only busy, but we were operating on a skeleton crew. Some clients walked in the salon at 8:30 pm, our regular closing time. This was the same time I thought I would have been walking out the door to attend church service. I ended up missing my plans for New Year's Eve church service. I was exhausted at the end of an unplanned double shift. I had not expected to be obligated the entire day. I finally arrived home, accepting the fact I missed New Year Eve's church service. Upon entering the house, I immediately began to escape the prison of my clothes with anticipation of a hot shower. Suddenly, the Holy Spirit prompted me to perform a breast exam on myself. I was prepared to shower and go directly to bed after my breast exam, but my discovery delayed my shower. I found myself staring in the mirror, wide awake. The possibilities of the hard rock I was feeling in my breast began to consume my thoughts. During my shower, I continued to press it. I eventually settled my mind around it being a lump, which could mean an early stage of breast cancer.

After dressing for bed, I laid there thinking and trying not to be in denial about what I had just experienced. I was holding on to faith and praying it was not cancerous. My mind was trapped between what the Word of God said about healing and the reality of the lump I felt in my breast. I was afflicted, to say the least. My original plan of sleeping was more like imagining myself laying on a cold doctor's table waiting for some dreaded medical results. I was completely numb. I had forgotten all about the stressful day I had encountered. I could not sleep so I stayed awake pacing the floor waiting for my family to return home from a New Year's Eve church service. Finally, I heard them at the front door. I didn't know how to break the news to my husband or my daughters who were fifteen, eighteen and nineteen years old at the time. Immediately, I pulled my husband into our bedroom to share the news of the lump. He performed another breast exam which unfortunately confirmed what I had discovered earlier. I had a lump in my left breast! We collectively decided we would not share the news with our daughters right away. We did not want to worry them prematurely.

I knew it needed to be examined by a doctor as soon as possible. We called my doctor's office and left a message requesting an appointment on the next business day following the Holiday. I suffered through the Holiday in silence. However, the alarm in my head would not stop ringing. I was devastated. So many questions and statements of my self-worth and identity consumed my thoughts all day:

"WHY ME?"

"WHAT DID I DO?"

"WHO DID I OFFEND?"

"I AM A PASTOR'S WIFE!"

"WHY IS THIS HAPPENING TO ME NOW?"

"I AM A WOMAN OF GOD WALKING BY FAITH!"

"I AM A GODLY EXAMPLE BEFORE MY CHILDREN!"

"I AM A FAITHFUL WIFE WHO LOVES MY HUSBAND!"

"I AM A PRAYING WOMAN OF GOD WHO LEADS BY EXAMPLE!"

I spent the entire Holiday silently repenting for everything I could think of, from my past to my present. Including speeding tickets, yelling at the dog and eating unhealthy foods. I was in mental anguish while waiting for New Year's Day to be over. I needed to put my anxiety to rest. I externally celebrated the day and the night time fireworks with my children, but internally I was a wreck.

Waiting to get an appointment scheduled and watching the clock tick down for the end of New Year's Day was like watching paint dry. It took what seemed to be forever. I anticipated that my doctor would reassure me, we had jumped the gun. I wanted to hear my doctor tell me the lump in my breast was a cyst or blackhead that just needed to be burst by a medical professional.

Thankfully, I was able to get an appointment the very next day after the Holiday. **Finally, it was the morning of my doctor's appointment.** My doctor confirmed I had a mass in my breast that required further diagnosis. She tried to comfort me when I became overwhelmed with emotions, but it did not work. She referred me to an Oncologist, but they did not have an opening on the schedule for two weeks. That was the most miserable two weeks I have ever experienced in my life. The thoughts in my mind during the waiting, ranged from me losing my life, to my husband getting remarried to a woman who would reap the benefits of the lifestyle God intended for me and I had contributed to through my career.

I fought off images of me lying in a casket. I had thoughts of me missing my baby girl's high school graduation. I thought about missing the wedding day of each of my three daughters and never meeting my future grandchildren. I even began seeking God about which friends I should ask to watch out for my daughters to ensure they would become successful Christian women.

I could not believe what was happening to me. My thoughts also included: Is it God's will to heal me or is this His way of transitioning me back to Him, in heaven. The struggle was real to stay confident and unwavering in what the Word of God states about being healed. The waiting and the battle raging in my mind was like hell on earth. It was awful. I often found myself balled up in a fetal position to try and escape the torment of my thoughts.

God's Handcrafted Thoughts

2 Corinthians 5:7 reminds us to walk by faith and not by sight. Sometimes this can appear to be an unrealistic task. But with God, nothing is impossible according to Luke 1:37. I encourage you to continue to walk out your life's journey with unwavering faith. No matter which health challenge you may be facing, walk by faith and not by sight.

Psalms 23:4 tells us that although we walk through the valley of the shadow of death, we should not fear because God is with us. We must be prepared to adjust to any life situation we face. We must strive daily to function at our highest level of faith even in the face of terminal illness.

Isaiah 54:17 declares that no weapon formed against us shall prosper.

Life Sustaining Scripture
Isaiah 55:11 So shall my word be that goeth forth out of my mouth; it shall not return to me void.

God's Handcrafted Affirmation
"God is Jehovah-Rapha, the Lord is my Healer."

CHAPTER 2

A Season in Life

My emotions took off like wildfire in a forest. I couldn't think or see straight after receiving the diagnosis. My feelings went from high confidence to a quick downward spiral. I felt like I was losing my mind. I lost focus at work, at home, in ministry and on what needed to happen just to make it through each day. I stopped serving in ministry. I did not want to pray for anyone. I even lost the desire to be intimate with my husband. My ability to function as a Proverbs 31 woman was losing its priority in my life since the diagnosis. Crying and devastating thoughts was my daily routine. The diagnosis was the first thing I thought of in the morning after a restless night. It consumed my thoughts twenty-four hours a day. I cried on the way to work and during my workday. I cried before and after servicing clients. I cried traveling to and from my destinations. Every time I found myself alone, I cried. I tried to make my main priority to remain sane and not give up on my will to live.

Despite my inward struggle, I also had to fight with the mask I wore for friends and family. They depended on me to be strong and function at the level they were accustomed. Another tough challenge was not sharing my health issue with close family members and friends. I chose not to share the news beyond my immediate family as lead by God. My total trust was in Him. My husband's desire was to let everyone know. I trusted God with all my heart and chose not to lean on my own understanding or desires. I had heard from God. I decided not to cancel out my faith in Him with negative conversations that could have resulted from sharing the diagnosis. No one except my husband, children, in-laws, a few friends like family and Pastor were aware of my diagnosis, until the day before the surgery. When my Pastor shared it with the congregation, which included my mother.

Leading up to the surgery, I struggled with the battle in my mind about dying and of God's ability to heal me. I was meditating and citing scriptures day and night. I believed the Word of God and was declaring it even within my mental struggle. I went a step further. Although I was a General Manager with a chain hair salon, I had the opportunity to assist clients as a licensed Cosmetologist. I received tips daily and made a conscious decision to take out my tithes every day, based on Malachi 3:11. I didn't want to make any mistakes about giving God what was due Him, according to scripture, in such an emotional state in my life. I remember a supernatural encounter with God that had the most significant impact on my mental fortitude. It was January 30, 2008. I had been crying nonstop for thirty days straight, and that was my thirtieth day. Amid my tears, the thought of how much I should give, to the church, as my tithes suddenly came to mind. It was around 6:30 in the evening and I was driving to pick up my second oldest daughter for Bible Study. I distinctly heard God's voice ask me a question. *"Why are you counting your tithes daily?"* In between tears, I answered God. *"I am taking out ten percent of my daily increase to give to you."* God asked me again, *"Why are you counting your tithes daily?"* My response this time was filled with attitude because the conversation was delaying my tears.

I was irritated at God for questioning my actions which were in line with His scriptures. I answered God, ***"Because I am commanded to give ten percent of my daily increase, and I want to be obedient!"*** He did not stop asking me questions despite my devout Christian response that lined up with the Word. God spoke to me again with a different question, *"What does it do for you?"* My response was, *"...according to the scripture in Malachi 3:11, you will rebuke the very devour for my sake."* Suddenly, my mind was free from the torment of the diagnosis and open to the emotional and physical healing of the Word of God. I had an epiphany through dialoguing with God. He would rebuke cancer for me. I would live and not die. I began to take authority over the diagnosis using the Word of God. It felt like fire alarms were going off inside of my spirit. At that moment, I was endowed with renewed strength that came from heaven upon me in what I can only explain as a supernatural experience.

I had received new revelation. I began to rejoice. I realized God was reminding me of His promises in Malachi 3:11 where it states: *"And I will rebuke the devourer for your sakes, and he shall not destroy the fruits of your ground; neither shall your vine cast her fruit before the time in the field, saith the Lord of hosts."* God immediately dried up my tears, and I took on the joy of the Lord as my strength. From that moment on, with boldness and conviction, I began declaring God's word over my life daily. I confessed God's word with divine authority and unwavering faith without failing. My healing confessions became my passion and reason for waking up every morning to connect with God. I believed without a shadow of a doubt that God's word would come to pass in my life. I was expecting God to perform a miracle and heal me.

God's Handcrafted Thoughts

Despite the doctor's diagnosis, we must take a righteous stand and confess the word of God with boldness, daily to receive the gift of healing. According to **Jeremiah 30:17** God has restored our health. Therefore, we must choose to walk by faith and not by sight. **2 Corinthians 5:7** Don't be moved by a diagnosis. **Isaiah 53:5** confirms that by Jesus Christ's stripes we are healed. Remember, almighty God spoke, and the heavens were created. You and I have been created in God's image. We can speak and confess the Word of God over our lives. When we speak the Word of God, we are releasing faith. Without faith, it is impossible to please God. **Hebrews 11:6**. Death and life are in the power of the tongue according to **Proverbs 18:21**. So, speak healing and stand on the Word of God in the face of your illness whether terminal or curable with medication. It is through the shedding of Jesus Christ's blood on Calvary that we are healed.

Life Sustaining Scripture
Malachi 3:11
"And I will rebuke the devourer for your sakes, and he shall not destroy the fruits of your ground; neither shall your vine cast her fruit before the time in the field, saith the Lord of hosts."

God's Handcrafted Affirmation
"I am blessed, and the Lord has taken sickness away from me."

CHAPTER 3

Strength to Believe

Out of obedience to God, I initially did not share the breast cancer diagnosis with anyone except my husband and daughters. This changed on the day that my middle daughter approached me with a revelation from God regarding who should know about the diagnosis. She was used by God to speak to me about how I was preventing our friends who are prayer warriors from interceding for me in prayer. I received the Word from the Lord through my daughter and shared the news of the diagnosis with prayer warriors that God laid upon my heart to intercede on my behalf.

Our Pastor was the first prayer warrior outside of my immediate family with whom my husband and I shared the news. He immediately prayed for me, the strength of our marriage and our children to endure through the season of my illness. God also lead me to share the diagnosis with Sister Owens who was also a prayer warrior. Not only had Sister Owens been a spiritual mentor in my life since the age of seven, but she had also been a Godly example for me as a wife and mother. I consider, myself to be her spiritual daughter and, in this season, she revealed through her actions, she felt the same way. She encouraged me and walked alongside me. God showed to me how Sister Owens was assigned to my life at a young age for this very season. She kept me sane when I felt like I was going to be lost in the distractions of what could happen other than God's promise of healing. I received the Word of God, with authority and conviction, through her every time she spoke into my life. I believed God, and I believed in what God was revealing through her even when the diagnosis said differently. She was my constant encourager during a season when I battled with being able to encourage myself.

My first appointment with the oncologist was scheduled for January 23, 2008. The anxiety I experienced during the waiting period included even greater mental anguish than what I had experienced before going to my first appointment following the discovery of the lump. The day I went to the Oncologist's office, my emotions were all over the place. I tried to be very strong, but the thought of the biopsy procedure caused me to become more and more overwhelmed with emotions. Even before a needle could penetrate my skin, I teared up with the thought of why they were subjecting me to such discomfort and pain. At 8:00 AM, I had an ultrasound. It was scheduled before I would meet with the doctor. The actual doctor's appointment was scheduled several hours after the ultrasound to give him time to receive the results. Although I knew this was all necessary, I did not appreciate the wait time between appointments. On the same day, I had to complete a biopsy procedure at 1:00 PM. I could not escape my new reality of doctor visits being an unsolicited part of my schedule. I was doing everything possible with my positive thoughts and prayers to keep my emotions in check while sitting in the waiting room. The wait time between 8:00 AM to 1:00 PM was my time to revisit my affirmations and stand firm on the Word of God. I was ready, or at least I thought I was prepared, to step down the hall leading to my biopsy room with confidence. I boldly sat in the waiting room imagining a bold and confident Cathy "Jewel" Chatman walking this day out with no tears.

I stood in victory from the chair that had been holding me as I waited. I took one step forward to walk the hall I had imagined myself walking down so many times in the five hours of waiting for my biopsy appointment. Suddenly, I felt a shift in my emotions as I strolled down the hallway toward the room where my biopsy would begin. My affirmations were a faint whisper in the back of my mind as I remember being overwhelmed with tears upon entering the room. Fear and every emotion possible overtook my body, and the strong woman I had just imagined, had left the building. I could not find her anywhere. I was left alone and crying a river as the procedure began. I tried, but I could not stop crying. I cried from the beginning to the end. My never-ending tears and emotions disturbed the medical professionals so much that I remember my husband being allowed to stand by my side even though we were initially told that he could not come in because it was a female only side of the office. My husband came in and tried his best to console me, but his presence did not stop the tears from flowing. My tears caused the seasoned technician to lose her composure.

My fear of the unknown was gripping me, the purpose of the doctor appointments, and the biopsy became my reality. I just needed to get through the moments of the day. I needed the needles to stop poking me and exchanging my peace for emotional outbursts that I could not control. I was stronger than this, is what I tried to say to myself, but I realized we are spirits having human experiences. I knew what to expect during the appointment because it was all explained. Nothing should have been a surprise. However, the warning of my emotional breakdown had not been disclosed and in the eyes of the medical professionals not expected. My imagination started going wild as I imagined the unknown possibilities of what would follow the biopsy. *"What will the doctor say now?"* *"How much worse could it be?"* The news of the diagnosis was bad enough. *"Could it get any worse?"* Before the first biopsy needle could penetrate my skin's surface, I begin imagining that I would bleed out and die even before the breast cancer could take me out. I started to imagine having a massive hole in my body which would be discovered during the tests. These thoughts gripped me with fear that tears were not enough to explain. I felt like a child having an adult nightmare in a world from which I could not awake.

I was overwhelmed with fear going into the biopsy. I kept imagining myself being a piece of meat poked, stuck and tenderized with a needle. After the biopsy procedure was complete, I must admit that all my anxiety was more of a distraction based on fear instead of faith. It was embarrassing and funny at the same time to realize that after all my crying and emotional outburst were done, I did not feel any pain. The nightmare I was living through leading up to the biopsy was meant to paralyze me in defeat versus trusting God for victory. I just needed the strength to believe the diagnosis was not unto death. My human experience caused me to be tossed to and fro in a sea of thoughts that created a false sense of reality. I sat there stunned and thought about how I emotionally affected everyone through the weakness I discovered when I failed to have the strength to believe.

I was told the results of my biopsy would be in on the next day. The next day came and went with no results from the doctor's office. When I did not hear from the doctor by 3:00 PM on the day following the biopsy, I was concerned. Finally, I took the initiative and called my doctor's office. However, the concern became a worry when I had not heard from the doctor in two days that turned to three days. By the fifth day, I was frustrated, to say the least, because I was not receiving a call back even after leaving countless voicemails. I was told that I would receive the results from the doctor or the nurse. Instead of me hearing from the doctor on the next day, it took five days before the doctor's office contacted me. During my five days of waiting, my thoughts started to drift back to the sea of negativity. I was more prepared for the thoughts that kept me emotionally unbalanced and in tears now, versus on the day I discovered the lump. I resisted the thoughts with the life-sustaining scriptures I was led to read. I also became inspired to write daily affirmations which helped me in my meditation and to combat the negative thoughts. The heavens opened when I finally connected with a live person on the phone, but it quickly ended in offense. Unfortunately, I had connected with a very rude nurse, and the only silver lining throughout the entire conversation was that she finally agreed to give a message to my doctor or his nurse stating I was urgently waiting to hear from them regarding the results of my biopsy. At this point, I was involuntarily participating in a waiting game that was out of my control. I had to employ reading scriptures and quoting affirmations to alleviate my frustration. The Word of God gave me the strength to believe and quieted the sea of negative thoughts.

My phone rang, and it was finally my doctor's voice on the other end. I was still working at the time. When the phone rang, I had just arrived home from work. I finally received the results of my biopsy. My family, my prayer warriors as well as myself were all praying and believing that the lump was just a benign tumor which would need to be surgically removed so that I could return to my life as usual. We were all ready for this season to be over so that things could get back to what we considered as our normal family life. The moment I heard the diagnosis I instantly thought about how one of my worst fears had come true. The doctor told me that I had Stage 1 breast cancer, but my lymph nodes were not cancerous. My doctor informed me that he would need to perform surgery immediately to remove the cancerous mass. We ended the phone conversation with my next appointment arranged for me to meet with him in person. Upon speaking to the doctor in person, my husband and I informed the doctor that we would be seeking a second opinion before setting a date for surgery. Unfortunately, my family life would never be what we considered to be normal again. God had a different journey for our family that included me being diagnosed with breast cancer. In the moments following the diagnosis, I remembered the night that I discovered the lump in my left breast and the morning that I shared the news with my husband as he arrived home from a New Year's Eve church service. Our strength to believe God would heal me began on January 1, 2008. When the doctor informed me that the diagnosis was breast cancer on January 28, 2008, our family realized that we would be facing a new normal that had to be rooted in our faith in the Word of God. We had to have the strength to believe that God would heal me and get the glory out of everything that we would face as the result of the diagnosis.

God's Handcrafted Thoughts

Despite what we may face in life, we must recognize that we are not alone. In the face of terminal illness, the devil tried to deceive me into believing that God had forgotten me and that I was alone. This was not true. I chose to believe the Word of God which states that God will satisfy us with long life according to **Psalm 91:16**. Therefore, we must remain steadfast in reading and declaring the Word of God. We must continue to enrich our lives by speaking what God has said about our healing through the scriptures. Always be mindful of what you speak. Words produce either negative or positive energy. We must exercise our faith by declaring God's Words consistently and without wavering. Our mindset about healing can only change by the confidence we display when we declare, believe and receive our healing. We must raise our faith to God's level of healing in agreement with what God has already spoken.

Life Sustaining Scripture
Psalms 91:16
"With long life will I satisfy Him and show Him my salvation."

God's Handcrafted Affirmation
"With long life will God satisfy me and show me His Great Salvation."

CHAPTER 4

God's Direction

I made the decision at the beginning of this journey not to tell my mother even though I knew it would come with future repercussions from my family. My mother was sitting in a church service on that Sunday when she heard the Pastor mention my name for prayer due to a surgery I had scheduled for Monday morning. Although he did not give any details, my mother immediately walked over to me, at the end of service, and asked why I was having surgery. I was faced with a direct question, and I did not want to lie in the house of the Lord. Therefore, I took a deep breath and *stated, "I am having surgery to remove breast cancer."* I felt a sense of relief and was comforted by being in a church service filled with the presence of God.

My mother left the service in tears with what I can only imagine was an overwhelming feeling of fear and hurt, because I never shared the news with her before that moment. Later I learned, she was devastated, and felt that the decision I made was very harsh. My husband also thought that it was the wrong decision. Later, I also found out she went to her brother's home immediately and shared the information with my family. Everyone was instantly upset about the diagnosis as well as me not sharing the news with my mom and other family members before the announcement in church. I received a phone call from my cousin expressing her concerns as well. Understandably, my cousin revealed that she felt I was wrong for not at least telling my mother. I would have never imagined that it would have taken over nine years for some members of my mother's family to recover from me choosing not to tell them. It took the death of a family member for us to reconnect and it was only because I was the person asked to contact everyone.

I honor her as my mother, but we have never had a very close relationship. Being an only child from a one parent home, I often spent my time alone and became withdrawn because of my height and insecurities. However, God's direction during that season was not to share what was going on with me with my mother. It was one of the most difficult decisions that I have ever had to make in my life. Several family members still have not spoken to me since that day. Now, my mother and I share a closer relationship. I knew I stood on the Word of God and followed the direction in which He led me, to not share the diagnosis beyond a select group of people. My obedience to God has allowed me to hold my first granddaughter in my arms and rock her to sleep. Even though I did not share my health issue with my mother and other family members, God led me to share the news with a select group of friends that are like family. During this time, I remember having an intense conversation with a dear friend. One of the things she said was my diagnosis was not unto death. When God used her to speak those words to me, they gave me life and freed me from my prison of mental anguish. She reminded me that if I did die, I was going to heaven to be with the Lord. So, it didn't matter what happened, because God had the power to heal me if He chose to do so. I remember her also stating that God was going to get the glory out of my life story. I celebrate now knowing the season of my diagnosis eventually caused me to experience a stronger bond with my mother than what I had experienced as a child.

Sister Owens was another friend who was like family and was a tremendous inspiration to me during that period. She was one of the first people, I shared my diagnosis with, outside of my husband and daughters. I have respected her as a Woman of God since I was seven years old. After I told her, we spoke daily. She was present for most of my doctor appointments. She covered me like I was her biological daughter. During our prayer time together, she sought the Lord on my behalf and asked Him Why would He let a young woman of God, with young daughters, so full of life, be diagnosed with a terminal illness? God responded to Sister Owens; He told her that my diagnosis was not for me. She always reminded me of what God had spoken. My experience with breast cancer was not for me. My experience was to bless someone else's life and draw them closer to God because of my testimony.

When I initially heard Sister Owens state my experience was to bless others, I didn't understand how God would possibly use my story for His glory. However, her words reminded me of my friend who stated, *"the diagnosis was not unto death."* Even though I was physically going through this encounter with a terminal illness, Sister

Owens and others consistently prayed with me and for me. This kept me focused on praying and meditating on the Word of God day and night. They helped me keep what I was going through in proper perspective. Despite the diagnosis, I was still blessed with my husband, daughters, and friends who loved me and trusted God to heal me. I also had God's promise that I would be healed for His glory and I knew my personal testimony would restore others for God's glory.

God's Handcrafted Thoughts

Because the power of life and death is in our tongues according to **Proverbs 18:21,** we must be very conscious of what words come out of our mouth daily. Our future is formed through the words that we speak. Strive to be diligent and speak healing into your life. Focus on what you speak and be intentional about what words come out of your mouth in all conversations. Be proactive. Know what you will say through your daily devotion and reading of the Bible so that you can declare what God says and not other's opinions. Preparation through reading and meditating on the Word of God is the key to overcome negative statements. Familiarize yourself with life-sustaining scriptures that reflect God's will for your healing. Embrace wellness in the face of an adverse diagnosis. Reclaim your longevity by declaring that you are healed.

Life Sustaining Scripture
Proverbs 18:21
Death and life are in the power of the tongue.

God's Handcrafted Affirmation
"The Lord gives strength to me and blesses me with peace."

CHAPTER 5

God Is a Strong Tower

G od's favor was with me. A close friend that I had not shared the diagnosis with called to say hello. While speaking to her, the Holy Spirit brought to my remembrance that she was a nurse with contacts at MD Anderson, the number one Cancer Center in the world. God lead me to share with my friend and share the challenges that I was facing as my husband, and I was seeking a second opinion regarding the diagnosis. Without hesitation, she became my ram in the bush and saved the day through her connections. Doors were quickly opened for me to set up doctor appointments. My struggle to connect with a doctor was over, but another unexpected obstacle lied ahead.

Victor and I decided for me to receive a second opinion from MD Anderson Cancer Center located in the Medical Center in Houston, TX. We did not know the decision to get a second opinion would also require us to make changes to our insurance network for me to have access to doctors at MD Anderson for the second opinion. Once all the changes were approved by our insurance company, which was thirty days after our initial decision was made, MD Anderson informed us that they did not accept our insurance provider. My patience was running thin, and only the prayers of my prayer warriors were quieting the storm that was beginning to rage in my heart. I rushed from doctor to doctor obtaining the necessary documents needed including additional x-rays which were required before meeting with an MD Anderson doctor for a second opinion. I was livid when I found out my insurance company had denied my planned appointments with a doctor at MD Anderson. I reached out to our insurance provider and found out that I needed to change my primary care physician under my insurance network to receive service. This was easier said than done and impossible since the arm of the insurance network that we were members of did not include MD Anderson as one of its service providers.

I could not believe that all my efforts and the willingness of the doctors to adjust their schedules to see me had abruptly come to a halt due to the doctors not being in the strand of networks approved by our insurance provider. I immediately began to pray. My husband and I had our sight set on me receiving a second opinion from doctors affiliated with the world renown MD Anderson hospital because we knew that they specialized in cancer treatment. We continued to keep hope alive, so I did not initially give upon finding at least one doctor within the MD Anderson network of doctors who would accept my insurance. After days of research, I found out that there were no doctors in the Medical Center that would take our medical insurance. We never imagined that obtaining a second opinion would cause us to face so many obstacles. I was sixty days into hearing the diagnosis that I had Stage 2 breast cancer. The rush to receive a second opinion was high on the priority list for my husband and I, but the obstacles faced due to insurance company changes caused time to continue passing, and my mind begin drifting back into the sea of thought that had previously caused me to cry rivers of tears. I continued to have the strength to believe that God is my strong tower. I pressed into God more and more and believed His Word that says, *"The name of the Lord is a strong tower and the righteous run into it and are safe."* Proverbs 18:10.

Prayer held my faith together and the sea of negative thoughts at bay as I began searching for a doctor to give us a second opinion within my network. I remember the night that I fell asleep crying after viewing the extended list of doctors included in our network. I was feeling overwhelmed and beat up emotionally. I had been so excited about my connection at MD Anderson being my solution for seeing a doctor sooner than later. I felt like I was on an emotional roller coaster ride. Spending additional time researching a doctor after the extended amount of time previously spent was not a task that I was looking forward to undertaking. I did not feel like I had the strength to start my research again. I remembered praying, crying and searching. My new job was praying, crying and searching daily because time was slipping away. I continued to think about the first doctor wanting to set my appointment for surgery immediately. At this point, we were over seventy days from the day that I received the initial diagnosis. God was my strong tower, and I ran to him to stay safe from the negative thoughts that were brewing in my mind. I begin to focus on what was going right and accepted the task of searching for a new doctor with the positive thought of at least the doctor is in my insurance provider's network. Finally, one day a physician's name seemed to illuminate on my computer screen. The name literally seemed to jump off the screen at me. After making an appointment as a new patient, I once again found myself in a position where I had to wait for the next available appointment on the doctor's schedule.

My first appointment with my new Primary Care Physician (PCP) was scheduled for March 12, 2008. I remember being scared but hopeful that the previous PCP's diagnosis could be wrong. I continued to trust God for healing and the possibility of the mass being benign. My new PCP met with my husband and I to confirm that the mass was not benign and what had previously been diagnosed with Stage 2 breast cancer was at a Stage 4 level. The breast cancer had spread to my lymph nodes. My new PCP immediately referred me to an Oncologist. Instantly, I received the referral, I realized God was in control of everything. The scripture Isaiah 55:8 tells us that God's thoughts are not our thoughts and God's ways are not our ways. Only God would have known after all my disappointment, I would be blessed to receive a referral to an Oncologist in the network we previously chose, after being denied by our insurance company. We were blessed to receive the insurance approved referral for an Oncologist who was formerly part of the MD Anderson Hospital network but was operating his own independent practice. Only God could have been working behind the scenes on my behalf to give me the desire of my heart related to who would provide me with a second opinion. God had redirected my footsteps, and I was reminded of the moment when I suddenly saw the name of my new PCP jump out at me from my computer screen. My family and I experienced Revelations 3:8 being manifested in my life. Yielding to God's will through prayer, I trusted God who is my strong tower. He closed a door to redirect me to His open door.

God truly showed Himself to be a strong tower at every turn in my journey even when I had done all that I could do. I praised God openly with verbal adoration. I knew without a shadow of a doubt God loved me so much He made a way out of no way. God removed me from the wait line the first day that I set foot in my new PCP's office. An appointment was arranged for me to visit the Oncologist on the next day before I left the office. Upon my first visit with the Oncologist, I was accompanied by Sister Owens and my husband. Reality set in. I received my third confirmation from the Oncologist that I not only had breast cancer, but I was at Stage 4 which was an even more severe diagnosis than my original Stage 2 diagnosis. How was this possible? I had to fight feeling angry with my insurance company for denying my previous attempts to see an Oncologist sooner. I became overwhelmed with emotions at the thought of the diagnosis being worse than initially stated. I found myself back in a place where I was emotional and crying as the negative thoughts started to flood my mind. I had been praying and believing that I would experience God's supernatural healing power and the lump would be miraculously removed. The instantaneous miracle which I believed God for, started to be poked with doubt when I realized that I was at a stage in the progression of the breast cancer when most people die.

The Oncologist who also performed my surgery to remove the cancerous lump carefully explained what I was going to be facing while on the operating table. The initial plan was for my left nipple to be removed for the Oncologist to have access to the lump. However, additional x-rays and Magnetic Resonance Imaging (MRI) images revealed that the position of the lump would require a left breast mastectomy. Again, I had to deal with the negative thoughts which accompanied my feeling of being mortal and this would be God's way of taking me from my husband and daughters. Anger mixed with being distraught is the best way I can explain my mental and emotional state while hearing the results. I lashed out at the doctor and told him that I didn't want to be mutilated. I was embarrassed, upset and filled with insecurities with the thought of my husband having to see me with one breast. What would be his reaction? Would he be as repulsed, as I felt like I would be, by living with a wife with one breast? The doctor could not hear the thoughts that were running through my head, but he heard my statement of not wanting to be mutilated.

The surgeon calmly and professionally responded that his intention was not to mutilate me. His plan was only to help save my life by removing the cancerous lump, and it would require me to have a mastectomy.

God's Handcrafted Thoughts

The rat race of our busy lives often appears to overtake us. We often fall prey to living a busy life which spirals outside of our control. The busy life that we have created becomes necessary to maintain our level of living. If we are continually doing the same ineffective things, we will not produce anything new in our lives. Let's change the course of our lives and exit the rat race which we have adopted in our lives as normal. We can do this by being willing and obedient to God, by believing God's Word and receiving the promises of our Lord and Savior Jesus Christ.

God is still in control even in the face of illness. Stand firm on the promises of God's word and declare the loving kindness of God every morning according to **Psalms 92:2**. We are children of God. Therefore, we should be led by the Spirit of God according to **Romans 8:14**. Cast all your cares upon Jesus Christ. **1 Peter 5:7**. Recognize that we are God's Hand-Crafted Jewels. Therefore, we are overcomers by the Blood of the Lamb and by the words of our testimony.

Life Sustaining Scripture
Psalms 107:20

"He sent his word and healed them and delivered them from their destructions."

God's Handcrafted Affirmation

"God sent His Word and healed me."

CHAPTER 6

Created in God's Image

Before I could get over the shock of being required to have my left breast mastectomy, I had to make my next appointment with the Plastic Surgeon who would do the reconstruction. As if having a mastectomy was not enough, I discovered during the appointment with the plastic surgeon I would be required to have my right breast reduced to match the implant that would be placed in my left breast during surgery. Nothing appeared to be getting better. Not only was I going to have to live with an implant in my left breast. I also had to deal with the loss of my bra's cup size which my husband had become accustomed to over twenty-four years of marriage. Suddenly, I had a choice to be confident in my appearance or be confident in the God who created me in His image.

I chose to be confident in the God who created me in His image. This meant I had to decide to choose life and not death. Without wavering, I decided to believe God would heal me. During my prayer time, God showed me He was my Jehovah-Rapha, in

Hebrew it means "to heal." God assured me He would take this sickness away from me according to Deuteronomy 7:15 and Exodus 23:25 which states:

Deuteronomy 7:15

"And the Lord will take away from thee all sickness,"

Exodus 23:25

"And ye shall serve the Lord your God, and he shall bless thy bread and thy water, and I will take sickness away from the midst of thee."

I put my faith into action when I informed each doctor at every level of my healing process that chemotherapy was not an option for me. Each doctor responded by saying, *"You will not survive without having chemotherapy."* It was the doctor's best medical opinion. In the eyes of the doctors, chemotherapy was the only option to kill all the cancer cells and keep the cells from forming in other parts of my body. To appease the surgeon and give my family peace, I reluctantly allowed a port to be placed in my right breast which would allow me to have chemotherapy after the surgery if I changed my mind.

Finally, the day of my surgery had arrived to remove the cancerous lump. April 24, 2008, is an anniversary date I would have preferred not to have but will always remember. My scheduled time to arrive at the hospital was 6:30 AM. The entire morning flowed like clockwork from my usual morning routine of prayer with God. He met me in my prayer time that morning and endowed me with His joy. I proceeded to get dressed and arrived at the hospital with my husband and in good spirits. My daughters were in school. However, a host of friends met us at the hospital. When we arrived to check in, the front desk informed us that we already had visitors. To our surprise, so many people met us at the hospital, the onlookers asked who I was in anticipation of a celebrity arriving. Hearing this gave me a reason to chuckle in the face of terminal illness and surgery that would change the outcome of my life. My husband stayed by my side until the intravenous fluids were hooked up in preparation for my surgery. I could feel the presence of the Holy Spirit with every step I took toward the operating table. Once the anesthesiologist arrived, and the tubing for anesthesia was inserted, I remember saying, "Ooh, this stuff really works. I already feel it traveling through my..." and that is the last thing that I remember before waking up in the recovery room. The surgery went smoothly. I was convinced before undergoing the procedure I would be healed in Jesus' name. I was ready to go through with the procedure, as a necessary process, to arrive at God's expected end for this season of my life, which would be total healing. No one from my mother's side of my family showed up on the day of surgery except my mother. As much as it saddened me that they did not show up or send me a get-well card, I stayed focused through faith and believed that one day they would forgive me. I trusted in God with all my heart and did not allow the feelings of disappointing my family to interrupt the positive affirmations and prayers I prayed leading up to the surgeries and I still pray now. I believed God knew what He had in store for me. Despite the emotional peaks and valleys, I experienced leading up to the surgery, it was a day of hope for me. I believed the prayers of the righteous avails much and knew that many positive prayers were touching and agreeing on behalf of my healing. I remember thinking a new horizon was opening for me, and I embraced the season as part of my destiny but not my destination. God's peace that surpasses all understanding overtook me and stayed with me during the surgery and remained with me through the reconstruction surgery.

God's Handcrafted Thoughts

Although we may experience life-altering situations, we must remember to renew our minds daily through the Word of God. It is vitally important to believe and receive healing when our life's journey includes a negative doctor's report. We should take on the mind of Christ according to **1 Corinthians 2:16**, we should call upon the name of the Lord and be saved. **Romans 10:13** says, just as we call upon the name of the Lord to be saved, we should also call upon the name of the Lord to be healed. To be healed by God, we should allow our minds to be transformed by the Word of God and not be influenced by the traditions of this World.

When chemotherapy was offered as the solution for me to be cancer free, I entertained the information against what I knew God had said to me. I realized after my decision that God had a handcrafted course of action, tailor-made for each of our lives.

However, God gives us a choice to choose his course of action or our own. **1 Corinthians 2:12** tells us that God has given us His spirit (not the world's spirit) to guide us into the free and wonderful gifts of grace and blessings. Our healing is a blessing.

Life Sustaining Scripture
Jeremiah 30:17a
"But I will restore you to health and heal your wounds."

God's Handcrafted Affirmation
"I meditate on His Word day and night."

CHAPTER 7

The Sea of Negative Thoughts

The peaceful moment before my surgery was interrupted by the hustle and bustle in the recovery room. I felt like it was more of a hurry up and wake up room. I spent about an hour there before being transitioned to a quiet hospital room. I did not wake up in heaven. Which was welcomed since I had faith for healing. I also wanted to see my daughters grow into successful women of God. As I opened my eyes to look around, I saw a glimpse of my husband, my oldest daughter and my mother waiting for me. As each one came to my bedside and gave me a hug, I purposely kissed each one of them. Their warm skin against my lips felt terrific, and I knew for sure that I was alive. Despite all the depressing disclaimers I had to sign related to what could go wrong during a surgery intended to save my life, my surgery went very smoothly according to the medical professionals. I did not experience any complications.

I spent eight glorious days in the hospital being waited on twenty-four hours a day by my group of angel nurses that took great care of me. The hospital felt like a safe place for me. I found myself dealing with anxiety and fear. When I thought of going back to my life away from the watchful eyes of nurses and doctors, my thoughts became focused on the life I formerly knew. However, God always made a way of escape through someone showing up in my hospital room with an encouraging word whether it was a nurse, doctor, friend or family member. I was still coming to grips with the drastic change that had occurred in my life. As I settled back into my life of taking care of my family as a wife, mother and daughter the sea of negative thoughts began flooding my mind like a cracking dam unable to bear the weight of the water. The enemy continuously tried to oppress and depress me through my thoughts. God showed me His love through people. Every need for encouragement and physical healing that I could think of God exceeded. All my needs were met.

During my recovery journey friends always seemed to know what I needed and when I needed it. One day, a friend stopped by to visit me in the hospital. I had suffered in silence with my thoughts and concerns following the surgery. God and I were the only ones who knew. I continued to project a positive, outgoing persona for family and friends. I was concerned about many things, but the most important at the time was not having the financial resources to give my baby girl her Sweet Sixteen Birthday Party. I considered this celebration an age milestone in a child's life. God sent a friend from church just in time this day. She stayed for hours. The Holy Spirit allowed me to share with someone for the first time about the thoughts which had become a burden during my time of recovering from surgery. I can genuinely say that the peace of God came into the hospital room that day as my church member ministered to me. By the end of our time together, I had cast all my cares upon the Lord. I was no longer concerned about how my husband and I would pay for my youngest daughter's sixteenth birthday celebration. I trusted her when she said, "Don't worry about a thing. It is already done."

My hospital discharge date was May 2, 2008. As much as I was not looking forward to my discharge date, I welcomed the thought of sleeping comfortably in my own bed next to my husband and having family time with my husband and daughters. I must admit, the days after leaving the hospital, I missed my group of angel nurses taking care of me. I was mentally prepared to go home following the mastectomy with the drainage tubes surgically placed in my body. However, my final checkup, before I was discharged, revealed I was healing better than the doctors had expected. The doctor surprisingly made the decision to remove my drainage tubes before I left the hospital. I smiled inside knowing God was keeping His promise to heal me. Not only was God healing me, but He was performing His promise quickly. Initially, my body was off balance from having the surgery so, I had to be assisted when walking to avoid falling. By my discharge date, God had blessed me to walk on my own, and I was feeling quite confident on my healing journey. The doctor continued to inform me that my recovery was not the typical results experienced by most patients. My body was recovering faster than expected. I gave God all the glory.

I walked out of the hospital and instantly remembered feeling the heat of the sun on my face. I was alive. That moment of feeling the warmth of the sun reminded me of when I woke up after surgery and felt the warmth of my family leaning in to hug and kiss my cheek as I opened my eyes. I did not imagine the transition between home and hospital would be so unusual. I had ridden in our car several times. However, this ride home felt like I was being transported by a rocket ship into outer space. My husband was not speeding but the forward motion of the car, at any speed, literally felt as if I was on a roller coaster ride or a passenger in a race car on a speedway topping at least 200 miles per hour. I had to hold onto the door handles just to endure the ride. I was awake, but my body was still recovering. I could not have predicted the unusual way my body responded to my ride home. However, I can say as the cliché goes my nerves were wrecked. We made it home safely, and my new life began the moment my husband opened the car door and helped me into the house.

God's Handcrafted Thoughts

God's word is more than a typical cliché. It exists so we may live a life full of everything we need, at all times. Although the trials and tests of life cause our attention to be focused on what we see and hear in our physical reality, the Word of God is still true. Be encouraged to know the Word of God brings complete wholeness which includes our physical healing. The motive of the devil is to steal our faith, kill our joy and destroy our life, but God sent His son Jesus Christ so we may have everything we need for an abundant life. **John 10:10** says God's purpose is to give us a full life full of all that we need. We are God's Handcrafted Jewels which means that we are made in the image of God. When our faith boldly declares God's ability, we are placed on God's winning course of actions for God's glory and our benefit.

Life Sustaining Scripture
Psalms 29:11
"The Lord will give strength unto His people. The Lord will bless His people with peace."

God's Handcrafted Affirmation
"God's Word is health and medicine to my mind, body, and soul."

CHAPTER 8

Fatal Consumption

P rior to discovering the lump in my left breast, my family was accustomed to planned meals which I cooked before I went to work. I was a regular gym participant. I also provided hair services for my own private high-end clients which included a National Basketball Association (NBA) Coach's wives. Life for me, my husband and children were nothing short of dreams coming true. I lost everything related to my hair career as the result of the diagnosis. I decided to focus more on my healing and trusted God for financial provision. Because of my mastectomy and cosmetic surgery, even standing in the kitchen to cook for my family of five was a difficult task. This disturbed my spirit because I believe in healthy food choices which resulted from me cooking for my family.

God answered my prayer. A dear friend went out of her way to make sure my family received a home cooked meal every Sunday during the month following my surgery. She was instrumental in coordinating the women of my church called the Elect Ladies to help her prepare and deliver Sunday home cooked meals to my family. The anxiety I felt leading up to the last days of my time in the hospital begin to turn into peace that surpasses all understanding. My hospital anxiety was due to the unknown life and lifestyle that awaited me after such a life-altering surgery and diagnosis. I lost my job and high-end hair clients, but I still had my family and my life. This reality was bittersweet, but I knew without a shadow of a doubt God was in control. My only responsibility was to trust God. Arriving home was a blessing. I experienced many gifts of love and thoughtful acts of kindness. People visited on a regular basis and encouraged us as a family and me individually. I needed it. I welcomed every positive thought, prayer and words that inspired me not to give up. I was also ensured that God had not forgotten me. Several times during my first few months home, I was comforted by words spoken to me in the hospital during the time I was concerned about celebrating my sixteen-year-old daughter's birthday. "It's already done." I can truly say that God is faithful to perform his word. I meditated on Philippians 4:19 daily, "But my God shall supply all your need according to his riches in glory by Christ Jesus."

May 6, 2008, was my first appointment after returning home from surgery. I had appointments with all my doctors, Primary Care Physician (PCP), Oncologist and Plastic Surgeon. My PCP's visit was a general meeting to confirm that my future meetings would be with the Oncologist because my PCP was not a Cancer specialist. The appointment with my Plastic Surgeon was to review my surgery and explain what I could expect in the healing process through my final results. I was also asked to commit to the multiple follow up appointments which would be ongoing for an extended period to monitor that I was healing according to plans. My final doctor's appointment for the day was with my Oncologist. I was not expecting what felt like an intervention from my doctor and nurse. Upon my doctor entering the examination room, his entire conversation seemed to be about why chemotherapy was the best preventive measure. No cancer was detected, but they recommended to all their patients to go through chemo to prevent the cancer from returning. The doctor and nurse convinced me that I would receive a very low dosage of chemo called a cocktail, and I would experience no drastic side effects. I eventually said yes to end the discussion and allowed the office to schedule my first of ten chemo treatments.

My first chemo treatment was scheduled for May 27, 2008. A dear friend agreed to get me to my first session so my husband would not have to continue missing work. It was very comforting to have her with me. During my first chemo procedure, I felt confident about what the doctor and nurse had explained. The low dosage cocktail appeared to be harmless. It felt like a standard intravenous drip given when a person is dehydrated. I left my chemo session feeling good. I was surprised the negative articles online did not prepare me for such a painless experience. My fear of the chemo treatment started to disappear after the first treatment. I confirmed my next doctor's appointment before leaving the office. The day after my initial treatment I was informed by my doctor's office that I needed to return to take a shot to increase my white blood cells. The therapy had gone so well with no noticeable side effects or pain,

I followed my doctor's request and went in for the shot. A different friend drove me to get the shot that woke up my entire body. The white blood cell shot took my pain level from zero to one hundred instantly. I did my best on the first day to tolerate the pain following the shot. By the second day, I found myself popping three Vicodin pills every two to three hours.

My husband noticed my speech was slurred and asked me how many pills I had taken. When he discovered I had not been waiting six hours between pills, he had me call my doctor's nurse who immediately requested that I be brought into the office for evaluation. Due to the number of pills I had consumed, no more time could be wasted in transporting me to the Emergency Room. The doctor decided to place me on an intravenous drip to flush the Vicodin out of my body. I was on the verge of a fatal over dose. That was day three. When I woke up with the memory of my near-death experience, I decided that I would not continue with the chemo treatment. As if the pain and almost fatal consumption of Vicodin were not enough on day four, day six following the chemo treatment brought its own horror. If I had not been convinced to stop taking treatments as the result of my day four experience, day six could have been the day I would have come to the same conclusion not to receive another chemo treatment.

On day six, following my first and only chemo treatment, I woke up feeling like hell's fiery furnace was located on the inside of my body. I was lifeless, sluggish and I could not find a comfortable position in which to sleep. Hot flashes, or as some call it personal summers, do not compare to the heat which I experienced for forty-eight hours. I could not see. I could not walk. I could not stand. I could not even sit. I was in constant torment. There was no comfort. The only comparison that came to mind was the torment of souls in hell for those who do not choose Christ as their personal savior. Thank God, I am a believer. I would not wish my experience on anyone including an enemy. Even when I somehow found myself drifting off to sleep, my body would jerk me awake uncontrollably. I felt like I was battling with a spirit of torment.

My thoughts went from disorganized to hallucinations. I lost my ability to see with or without my glasses. It was the worse feeling of my life. My mind was in such dismay I could not find the words to pray more than *"Father help me!"* When I could get my thoughts in order, I focused on talking to God, and I remember telling the Lord if He would allow me to come out of this, I would not return to another chemotherapy session or be subjected to another white blood cell shot. Instead of seeking God's voice for chemo treatments, I allowed the doctor and nurse to convince me to go against God's first direction. If I had any doubt of being out of the will of God, I knew that my current state of agony was not the will of God for my life.

God's Handcrafted Thoughts

When walking through the emotional and physical journey of dealing with a terminal illness diagnosis, it can feel like you are going through hell on earth. However, God is in control no matter what you may face in your life. Recognize that it is not the end of your life's journey. Using faith filled words daily such as "the Lord will deliver me from every evil work" creates the blessed life that God has promised us. Faith filled words are our weapons to deliver us from every evil work. God's Handcrafted Affirmations found at the end of each chapter in this book are examples of faith filled words. Declaring these words daily will help activate our faith and allow God's blessing of healing to be manifested in our lives. We will experience daily victories through our words despite our illness. Our words are powerful. Our words carry either faith or fear. Choose words that carry FAITH even in the face of terminal illness.

Life Sustaining Scripture
2 Timothy 4:18
"And the Lord will deliver me from every evil work and preserve me for His heavenly kingdom. To whom be glory forever and ever. Amen"

God's Handcrafted Affirmation
"I am delivered from every evil work and my life is preserved for God's kingdom."

CHAPTER 9

Lymphedema

Months after my surgery I felt great and wanted to get back into the groove of things, work-wise. I felt as though I could pick up where I left off before the mastectomy. After surgery, I was advised not to lift over 25 pounds and to avoid overexerting my body. So, I searched for career opportunities that fit the criteria given to me. I thought of seeking a career as a chauffeur. So, I researched and pursued the opportunity. We had a friend that was a chauffeur and gave me all the information I needed. Venturing into becoming a chauffeur became a gratifying career. I imagined being fitted for my new black suit and the black patent leather shoes to accommodate the look.

Going to work and meeting people with various lifestyles and careers was enjoyable. The income was what I wanted. Chauffeuring was a dream job. I had opportunities to meet celebrities, music legends, Millionaires and CEO's of major companies. Weeks went by before I noticed a change in my body. I started experiencing swelling and discomfort in my upper left arm. It became a regular part of my day as a chauffeur. One thing I did not prepare for was lifting luggage and heavy bags as I continued to heal. I assumed the lifting would not be an issue, but as I zeroed in on what was causing the pain, I decided to stop my career as a chauffeur.

We needed two incomes in our household, so I began to pray for the next opportunity that would be a good fit for my altered lifestyle. Shortly after making the decision to stop working as a chauffeur, I received an unexpected phone call from a friend who owned her own business and needed assistance. She was looking for someone to be an Event Coordinator for a senior property her company was managing. I interviewed for the position and got it. The job description was ideal to accommodate my physical requirements after surgery. It was a rewarding assignment. I enjoyed going to work every day. The daily tasks were unique. There was never a dull moment. One task was to drive the seniors to the grocery store weekly. It was something they enjoyed. Getting out and being independent. Sometimes I would help those that were disabled and couldn't lift their bags. We even ventured out to the movies and to lunch monthly.

Over time, I began to feel another change in my body. Again, I started experiencing swelling and discomfort in my upper left arm. I also noticed redness and pain in the area, which was a sign of inflammation. Because I enjoyed what I was doing at the senior property I ignored the symptom as the days, weeks and months passed. The symptoms began to increase with discomfort. I started to experience numbness in my left hand. My left arm would swell and throb daily. I was afraid and began to worry. As I continued my daily activities the symptoms increased and began to alter my personality.

While driving at work, my entire upper left side would go numb. I didn't know what to think or do. After six months of unbearable pain, I made a doctor's appointment to get checked out. My primary care physician began to run all kinds of tests, and the tests would come back normal. I would go back to my daily routine. And the same issue would continue to present itself. Numbness, swelling and discomfort in my upper left arm. I didn't know what to do. I was scared and didn't know who to confide in. My doctor's appointments became a part of my weekly calendar. I was concerned that I was having a stroke and it was going undiagnosed. The discomfort and the change in my body could not go undetected anymore. My life had taken a whole new tailspin. I was confused because I was walking in the healing that was prophesied to me. I couldn't understand what was happening. I was happy in my new career path. My family life was thriving. My career was exciting, and I was walking cancer free. Worry, frustration and fear began to escalate. Week after week, the pain increased. I lost my focus at work, and the discomfort in my body started to affect me.

My primary care physician had exhausted all her means and began to refer me to specialists. A cardiologist was one of the specialists recommended, based on the symptoms I was experiencing, but we hit a dead end. That physician couldn't help me. However, he listened to me very carefully and was able to appropriately refer me to a neurologist. **Bingo!** This was the winning moment in time. It was six months later; entering the Christmas

Holiday. I had come to a conclusion; if I had not received any results by the end of 2009, I was going to check myself into the hospital and remain there until someone could tell me what was happening to my body.

Before leaving for Colorado for Christmas, I had my first appointment with the neurologist, who became my new best friend. As I described the symptoms, I was experiencing the neurologist understood what I was describing in my body. He said you have LYMPHEDEMA. And I said, *"what is that?"* He began to explain to me what lymphedema was. It is swelling in an arm or leg caused by a lymphatic system blockage. Secondary lymphedema occurs because of an obstruction or interruption that alters the flow of lymph through the lymphatic system and can develop from an infection, cancer, surgery, or trauma. People who have had a simple mastectomy, in combination with axillary (armpit) lymph node removal, experience lymphedema. My neurologist went on to explain that Lymphedema can occur within a few days, months, or years after surgery. A small amount of swelling is reasonable for the first four to six weeks after surgery. I began to weep uncontrollably. I couldn't believe that it took six months for someone to finally correctly diagnosis me.

My mind went out on a wild imaginary ride. Finally, I was relieved. The fear of having a stroke or heart attack diminished. My neurologist explained to me that I would be referred to the Lymphedema wound care treatment center where I would be able to receive further care and get the symptoms under control. After having my first consultation, I was made aware that it was a three-month commitment to the lymphedema wound care center. That was the minimum time it would take to stabilize my body. The most important aspect of treatment was learning how to care for my health. My family and I were educated on how to maintain treatment at home. Turning in my resignation was a tough decision to make, but overall, I was relieved. At that moment all I could do was give God the praise, glory, and honor that was due Him.

I was back to square one. After receiving this information, I decided to stop working as the Event Coordinator and focus on getting well. I would have never imaged that a mastectomy would cause this much damage to my body. I learned that Lymphedema develops after breast surgery because there is an alteration in the pathway that drains the fluids involved in the immune system. It can occur at any time after the surgery. If untreated, it can become worse, which is what happened to me when I attempted to return to work. The decision to stop working put a strain on our finances again. A two-income household is a must in today's economy. But, I decided my health was more important than a career or money.

Deciding to stop working was a huge step for my family and I. It caused a ripple in my marriage. For the first time, I faced the fact I would be disabled for a period. I was led to apply for my disability. It took forever to be approved and begin receiving income to help with our monthly expenses.

God's Handcrafted Thoughts

When we are faced with an outward appearance of a physical or diagnosed disease. We must believe even more what God has promised in His Word. **Exodus 23:25** delivers a promise to us, God said he would TAKE sickness away from us! Take is an action word. It means God is moving on our behalf. It is imperative that we believe and receive the Word of God.

Exercising our faith according to **Hebrews 11:1**, *Now faith is the substance of things hoped for and the evidence of things not seen.* Now is defined as the present time. God is consistently moving on our behalf. And we must choose to walk by faith daily. Join in with me and Thank God for baring our sicknesses and diseases in His body on the tree; *by his stripes WE ARE HEALED!* According to **1 Peter 2:24.**

God's Handcrafted Affirmation

"I am blessed, and the Lord has taken sickness away from me."

Life-sustaining scripture

3 John 2

"Beloved, I wish above all things thou mayest prosper and be in health even as thy soul prospereth."

Life-sustaining affirmation

"I walk in total health and complete wholeness."

CHAPTER 10

Eat to Live

After my diagnosis, it became even more critical that my eating lifestyle lined up with God's will for my life. I became laser-focused on my dietary choices. My significant research and investigation on what causes cancer, helped me conclude that our diet intake was vital. A plant-based diet was made very apparent to me. I began to understand our bodies were made to heal itself. I also found eating right for my blood type was vital. *What I am now sharing is solely based on a personal decision.* I read cancer can't survive with oxygen. So, I began my mornings by inhaling deeply and exhaling. I found this will get the oxygen flowing in my red and white blood cells and causing my lungs to operate at their optimum level. Also, cancer can't survive in a body that is alkaline. Chronic disease cannot take root in a body that has a well-balanced PH. Which means the PH of your body is in a more alkaline state, rather than the acidic state. The body is always trying to maintain equilibrium at a pH of 7.365, which is slightly alkaline (*Dr. Axe food is medicine*).

A 2012 review published in the Journal of Environmental Health found that balancing your body's pH through an alkaline diet can be helpful and the key to longevity and fighting chronic disease. I chose to eat fresh fruits and vegetables daily. Vegetables and fruits help me sustain a healthy lifestyle. Some vegetables have carotene to help increase the number of infection-fighting cells. Sometimes I ate frozen foods accompanied with unprocessed plant-based sources of protein. Which helps to protect my healthy cells and balance essential mineral levels. Always consult with your primary care physician before beginning any healthy lifestyle changes. Listed are some healthy tips:

- Strive to reduce foods high in salt and fat.
- Eat a variety of foods to get all the nutrients you need.
- Drink plenty of water - Drinking **Water** Helps Maintain the Balance of Body Fluids. Your body is composed of approximately 60% **water**. The functions of these bodily fluids include digestion, absorption, circulation, creation of saliva, transportation of nutrients, and maintenance of body temperature.
- Maintain your ideal body weight. A registered dietitian or your health care provider can help calculate your ideal body weight.
- Always check with your doctor first before starting a new exercise program.
- Exercise regularly

During and after my diagnosis I increased my daily devotions and affirmations that lined up with the word of God concerning health and healing. I would thank God for healing my body of cancer. I would confess that sickness and disease (cancer) had no place in my body. I would put God in remembrance of his word.

Hebrews 13:8 says, Jesus Christ is the same yesterday, today, and forever.

Ecclesiastes 7:17 asks *"Why should I die before my time?"*

Usually, when you receive a diagnosis of cancer, you immediately think of death. But Psalm 118:17 became my best friend; *I shall not die but live and declare the works of the Lord.* So, overcoming fear and choosing to walk in divine health became my banner for my life. Because God had not given me a spirit of fear, but of power, and of love, and of a sound mind according to 2 Timothy 1:7. I embraced when God said to me that he has restored my health and healed me of cancer according to Jeremiah 30:17.

CHAPTER 11

Total Confirmation

Three weeks had passed, and it was June 16, 2008, which was the day of my next scheduled chemo treatment.

After going through my experiences following my first treatment, my mind was made up. I was not going to subject myself to another chemo treatment and be disobedient to God's first instruction which was not to have chemo treatment. I was not going to argue with God because the physical results following my first chemo treatment was all I needed to be convinced that the small dosage cocktail was not God's will for my recovery process. Even though I informed the doctor I was not going to schedule any additional chemo treatments, I followed his request for me to have blood work done. The results of the blood work came back on June 17, 2008, and I am sure the doctor expected the results to be his support as to why I should agree to another treatment. However, the blood work proved that my red blood cells were too low for me to receive chemo treatments. The result of my bloodwork was my final confirmation I did not need another chemo treatment. I took my final stand against chemo treatments that day. I walked out of the doctor's office proclaiming my healing and went to my holistic doctor the same day.

Faith in the face of a terminal illness took root over time. I had to shift my thinking from man's traditional cures and chemo treatments to God's alternative healing methods. I was recommended to a holistic doctor through a divine appointment. Several months before discovering the cancerous lump, I met a woman who not only became a hair client she also became a good friend. While in conversation with her many times before the breast cancer diagnosis, she mentioned her holistic doctor and he is the one that I went to the day I walked out of my doctor's office. When I was faced with the decision of continuing chemotherapy or being obedient to God and canceling additional sessions, the Holy Spirit reminded me of what my hair client had shared about her holistic doctor and her holistic lifestyle.

The knowledge was great and received, but I did not recognize God was calling me to embrace a holistic lifestyle through what appeared to me as a casual conversation. Suddenly, God brought back the conversation with my client as His solution for me to heal supernaturally from the diagnosis of breast cancer. My faith believed that God could heal me through a holistic lifestyle even when, so many others chose the traditional paths. I knew if I were going to trust God and choose a holistic lifestyle, I would need to hear God's voice and silence the opinion of everyone who I loved and who loved me. Fear was my biggest enemy to hearing God. I found myself fighting fear with faith for many days following my decision to discontinue chemo treatments. I fought fear with faith in the face of a terminal illness. Some days my faith may not have been as strong as others, but I practiced my faith. I created morning times with God when I would be lead to scriptures which I would meditate on throughout the day. Every morning I would wake to the Holy Spirit giving me a fresh word that affirmed my faith straight from God's lips to my ears. These words became my God handcrafted affirmations. I would then end my time with God every morning by writing down the thoughts which were crafted during our time together. This morning devotional time became part of my life's routine for building my faith in the face of a terminal illness.

I now know God brings people into our lives to accomplish His plan and purpose for our lives. The contribution from people God divinely appoints in our lives can be through a word of encouragement, unsolicited information, transportation or even the hands that cook a hot meal for my family when I was not able to stand. God prepared my life for the journey which I did not see coming. He had already gone through so He could direct my path of healing. His thoughts are not our thoughts. I thought my faith was as strong as any other believer in Christ. That was what I believed before the journey of God healing "Jewel" physically, mentally, emotionally and spiritually. I never realized God's way of allowing me to embrace a new level of faith would come through the diagnosis of breast cancer. My first step to reclaim my longevity and embrace wellness, my first step was to fully trust God beyond what I could control or understand. Not leaning on my own understanding was the only option. It was a mandate. It was a requirement for me to receive the supernatural healing God had promised me and had confirmed through others. I could not waiver in trusting God with ALL my heart. Having faith in this time was not easy. This decision meant that I had to stand up to feelings of fear, loneliness, restlessness, depression, oppression, low levels of energy, and days of feeling ill. Each good or bad day physically, I had to stand up for my decision not to take any additional chemo treatments or immune system shots. I had to trust God and have faith beyond measure.

I started my holistic lifestyle journey on June 17, 2008. To begin my holistic lifestyle journey that would change my life, my first step was to eradicate the toxins that were tormenting my body. The holistic doctor confirmed my system was very toxic through my blood work. At this time, my faith that a holistic doctor could impact my healing was based on obedience to God and an unwillingness to subject my body to the symptoms that followed by chemo treatment. I must admit my decision to trust God was more important to me than my belief that a holistic lifestyle would be necessary for God to perform His supernatural healing. During my consultation with my holistic doctor, he assured me he would be my Holistic Coach through my healing process. He walked me through my health improvement program which included my dietary guidelines and nutritional supplements. I expected the medical terms and professional interpretation of my current and future medical condition. However, I was not expecting my holistic doctor to be a Holy Spirit lead believer in Jesus Christ just like me. My spirit leaped inside me when the doctor reassured me that my healing would come not only through my dietary guidelines and nutritional supplements, but my healing would also occur through God's healing powers invading my mind, body, and soul in response to my spiritual commitment to God.

Before my first chemo treatment, I was leaning on my own understanding and miseducation received through medical marketing about cancer and the importance of chemo treatments which I had grown up hearing my entire life. When my Holistic Doctor acknowledged his faith in God while providing me my bloodwork diagnosis, I knew I had made the right decision to trust God and discontinue my chemo treatments. I became a willing and obedient patient. God was able to use my holistic lifestyle and the doctor, who also believed in Him, as the alternative method of healing my body.

God's Handcrafted Thoughts

When we are faced with a terminal illness diagnosis, we should immediately begin meditating and declaring **Ephesians 6:10-15**, *"[10] Be strong in the Lord and in His mighty power. [11] Put on the full armor of God so that you can take a stand against the devil's schemes. [12] For our struggle is not against flesh and blood but against the rulers, the authorities, against the powers of this dark world and against the spiritual forces of evil in the heavenly realms.[13] Therefore, put on the full armor of God, so that when the day of evil comes, you may be able to stand your ground, and after you have done everything, to stand. [14] Stand firm then, with the belt of truth buckled around your waist, with the breastplate of righteousness in place, [15] and with your feet fitted with the readiness that comes from the gospel of peace."*

We should also meditate and declare that God is our strong tower found in **Proverbs 18:10**. Our faith can often be tested by the demands of life, but we should not fail to stand on scriptures and declare that we are healed according to the Word of God.

Life Sustaining Scripture

Ephesians 6:10

"Finally, my brethren, be strong in the Lord and the power of His might."

God's Handcrafted Affirmation

"I am strong in the Lord and in the power of His might."

CHAPTER 12

The Many Breasted One

O n Wednesday, June 18, 2008, I woke with a spirit of expectation and excitement. I was excited about the opportunity to be in church for the second time since my surgery. I arrived at the church service with a spirit of expectation. The praise and worship did not disappoint me. I felt the presence of God through the praise and worship experience. We had a guest speaker. I remember him having white hair like I imagined Moses did when he came off the mountain after experiencing God through the burning bush. He was a Prophet of God and a Pastor. God's anointing was upon him, and I witnessed the power of God like never before. During the church service, I watched as people were miraculously healed. People who had no fillings suddenly had gold and silver fillings in their mouth. People testified of having miraculous weight loss during the service. Everyone honored God and testified to the power of God performed miracles. During the service, the Prophet announced, *"A woman is being healed of breast cancer, and she will experience growth where her surgery was performed."* I immediately received the Word of God from the Prophet. My husband and several friends also heard the same declaration and received the Word of God from the Prophet for me. I begin to believe my healing was done in Jesus' name. I started celebrating my healing upon receiving the Word of God. Throughout service, I kept looking for the miracle. Although the miracle did not manifest during service, I never doubted the power of God. I kept on praying and confessing the Word of God over my body daily. I continued to anoint my body with blessed oil and kept believing the words of the Prophet.

My left breast was flat as my chest after the mastectomy, but my faith did not waiver. Even when the physical manifestation did not occur the same night or the next day, I continued to believe the words spoken by the Prophet. When I woke on the morning of June 24, 2008, I woke later than usual and missed my morning devotion time with God. I remember heading straight to the shower and performing my daily faith check for a growth in my left breast. This morning was different. There was growth just like the Prophet stated on June 18, 2008. Eventually, I discovered that my new left breast bra size was a size A cup. This was indeed a miracle, and I was in total awe. Six days after I received God's prophetic word from the Prophet, the prophecy had manifested in my physical body. I experienced growth in the place where the left breast of my mastectomy had occurred. I instantly began leaping and praising God for the miracle I was experiencing. I was amazed. I became overwhelmed with joy. Words can't express a moment that is personal between God and me. At that moment, I knew Jewel was not just my middle name.

I felt like *a priceless Jewel handcrafted by God.* The miracle of the growth in my left breast was not the only miracle that manifested from the words spoken by the prophet. The Prophet also stated people would experience dental work and would receive gold and silver tooth filings with doves and crosses on them. I quickly ran to my vanity to look in the mirror for my second miracle. There it was. I suddenly saw three silver filings with crosses on the right side of my mouth which were not placed there by a dentist. My dentist fillings were on the left side of my mouth. I believe that my three fillings represented the father, son and Holy Spirit. This is the day that I believe God's supernatural healing took place in my body and the signs and wonders I experienced that day were God's assurance my healing was complete. Mark 16:17 states, *"And these signs shall follow them that believe."* I ran to show my husband and daughters who were at home at the time. Everyone began to rejoice. My middle daughter started running and praising God for the miracles. My youngest daughter started shouting and praising God.

After sharing the news of God's miracles with my family, I begin to call every friend that came to mind who had walked with me through my journey from the day of the cancer diagnosis to the day of my supernatural healing. I also called my Pastor, and he began to praise God. One of my dear church friends who is also a Registered Nurse immediately jumped in her car and came over to witness and celebrate God's miracles with my family and me. I was not ashamed to show anyone who walked through the door the miracle that God had performed in my left breast and in my mouth. My family and friends continued to marvel at the work of our Lord and Savior Jesus Christ of Nazareth.

The next day, after the physical manifestation of my miracles spoken by the Prophet, was Wednesday, June 25, 2008. It was the Wednesday night service immediately following the Prophet's visit. My Pastor allowed me to give my testimony during service. People in the service instantly started rejoicing and even leaping over chairs in excitement and praise. It was an explosive night of celebrating the goodness of God and His healing power. People raised their voices in victory, shouted, cried and even ran the length of the church. Wednesday night was an unplanned night of praise. The Pastor did not deliver his planned message. He gave over to the celebration of God brought on by my testimony and God using it as a platform for His glory. The service was live streamed which enabled my testimony to be broadcast worldwide.

The immediate Friday following my Wednesday night testimony, I found myself in a place of shame. My day started off with my morning meditation, and I was still basking from the presence of God that filled the room following the delivery of my testimony. I was excited about an opportunity to attend a special event meeting for my church that was scheduled at a restaurant later that day. I decided to prepare myself for the meeting sooner than later so I would be on time when my ride to the meeting arrived. I decided to shampoo my hair to prepare for the meeting. I had the perfect clean and cute hairstyle in mind for the evening. As I shampooed my hair to my surprise, it appeared to be shedding. I initially did not become alarmed. However, shedding transitioned to clumps of hair literally falling out into the sink. The more I shampooed my hair, the more hair ended up in the sink. I could not believe what was happening. I stood over the sink with my hair in my hands. My heart sank. I could not think passed the bald image that was staring back at me in the mirror.

Discouragement began to seep into my emotions, and I started to weep and yell uncontrollably. I felt hurt and betrayed by my doctor and his nurse who told me that the low dose chemo treatment cocktail would not have any side effect. I was confused by the information shared about the treatment and the results that I was experiencing. I was stunned and pacing the floor. My thoughts went back to the first day I discovered the lump to the chemo treatment and the recent word of the Prophet. I tried to call my husband, but he was busy at work. So, I reached out to a close friend to confide in about my hair loss experience. I was crying to a point where she could not understand what I was trying to tell her. She was totally caught off guard. She began to pray with me. I eventually spoke to my husband while he was at work. When he came home from work, he saw me and did not show any emotions. He was very comforting and helped me shave my head, and he shaved his head as well. My husband and I talked and prayed together. At this point, my spirit rested. I became calmer than I had been all day and I received peace from God. I felt embarrassed by my hair loss. I was ashamed of my baldness and did not want to go to the meeting. God had other ideas. After I came to myself, God dried my tears. I received the direction from God to go to the meeting. God lead me to choose a wig from the collection of wigs that were already in my possession. I attended the meeting as planned. Even though no one could see under my wig, I still felt self-conscience. I kept being concerned about my wig falling off at any moment and I did not want anyone to know that I was completely bald since the wig had nothing to cling to. Every time I walked, I could feel the wig shifting.

The day after experiencing my hair falling out, I began to receive calls of encouragement. Members of my family had shared the news with friends. Many friends came over to support me with words of encouragement, hair products, and accessories to assist me in covering up my baldness. God gave me beauty for ashes. I became excited by the different styles and fun colors that were gifts to help me with another phase of my healing journey. I was even blessed with lace front wigs. I reclaimed my confidence by the end of the day on Saturday. The enemy tried to steal my joy. The devil thought he had my thoughts, but I took on the mind of Christ. I declared I am an overcomer by the blood of the lamb and the words of my testimony. The first six months of 2008 seemed like the longest time of my entire life but the most rewarding time of my life as well. My faith was challenged, but it grew in ways I did not realize was required by God. There were days I found myself confused and disconnected from people and from God. Through the process of healing, I doubted I would arrive at a place where I could rejoice in God's supernatural healing.

At the end of my physical healing process, I realized I was called and chosen by the Lord for the season I experienced. God chose me to be healed supernaturally because he knew He could trust me to give Him the glory. No one else in my family had experienced a breast cancer diagnosis. There was no history, from which the doctors could pull information. The day I experienced growth in the left breast where the doctor had performed my mastectomy I felt loved and validated by God. I am so proud to share my testimony of God's supernatural healing of my body with signs and wonders.

Although I am less one natural breast, which was replaced with an implant after I experienced growth to a size A cup, I acknowledge my Lord and Savior Jesus Christ who is the many breasted one for our lives. My awareness of who God is through my experience of being diagnosed and then of being healed supernaturally from breast cancer has me feeling more beautiful now than I ever did before with two proportioned breasts. I literally feel sexier than ever. I am more confident, and I know who I am in the Lord without wavering. I am God's, Handcrafted Jewel. I have accepted my call to be an Evangelist that shares the news of God's supernatural healing power. My new life's purpose is to inspire people to embrace wellness and reclaim their longevity in the face of a terminal illness through their faith in God. He is able to supernaturally heal sickness, deliver from depression and set free a mind captive by negative thoughts.

I still meditate daily on God's life-sustaining scriptures. I continue to boldly declare God's handcrafted affirmations over my life, and I continue to document God's handcrafted thoughts which are downloaded each time I meet with him for my morning devotion. I stand in faith and in God's supernatural healing power. If I had 10,000 tongues, I could not completely express my gratitude to God for the miracles that I have experienced on my life's journey. It feels like my longevity multiplies every time I share my testimony. God has been better than good to me.

God's Handcrafted Thoughts

El-Shaddai means God Almighty. During my time of being diagnosed with terminal illness, God revealed to me He is the many breasted one. God shows us his perfect love and reminds us of the sufficiency we have in Him. He has provided each of us His devotion, love, and loyalty in abundance. God's abundant blessings are poured out on our lives daily. **Psalms 115:14** declares God shall increase us more and more. God will cause us to flourish and thrive in the ways of the Lord. We are blessed of the Lord which made heaven and earth. **Psalms 115:15**. God blesses us to prosper in every area of our life. So, it is possible for us to embrace wellness in the face of a terminal illness. It is also possible for us to reclaim our longevity by declaring, believing and receiving our healing through the Word of God which has already been spoken.

Life Sustaining Scripture
Isaiah 58:8a
"Then shall thy light break forth as the morning, and thine health shall spring forth speedily."

God's Handcrafted Affirmation
"Daily my light breaks forth like the morning and daily my health springs forth speedily."

ABOUT THE AUTHOR

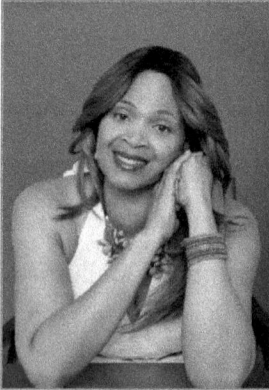

Cathy "Jewel" Chatman surrendered her life to Christ as a child in 1974 and rededicated her life to Christ as an adult in 1982. She has been faithful to the House of God for over forty-five years. As an Ordained Minister, Jewel has served in various ministry leadership roles including but not limited to the Marriage Ministry, Elect ladies, Bible exhorters, Children and Youth Ministries and Event Ministries. She has also served as a mentor in the Harris County Public School System and Vice President for So Blessed To Be Me, Inc. Board of Directors (www.blessedtobeme.org). Jewel is also the Founder of Cathy Chatman Ministries in Houston, TX.

Jewel has been a dedicated wife to her husband Victor for over thirty-five years. She is also the mother of three beautiful daughters. Tiffany, Victoria, and Danielle are all adult women honoring Christ with their lives. And a grandmother to her first granddaughter Aria Michelle. Jewel has also impacted the lives of over fifty motherless and inherited children for Christ as a Foster Care Mother.

In addition to being a committed wife and mother, serving in ministry and volunteering her time to mentor girls, Jewel has been a successful entrepreneur in the beauty, health and wellness, and legal services industries for over twenty-five years. However, Jewel contributes her most significant life accomplishment to God. Jewel's faith grew to levels not previously experienced as she deployed her faith in Christ and the Word of God as her weapon against Stage 4 Breast Cancer. Jewel won the victory in Jesus' name and has been a Stage 4 Breast Cancer Survivor for over ten years.

To invite "Jewel" to be a Guest Speaker at your next meeting, event or conference, email cathyjewelchatman@gmail.com.

To learn about Jewel's upcoming events and to become a Jewel Insider go to bit.ly/godshandcraftedjewels.

Jewel hosted the first God's Handcrafted Jewels Women's Retreat in Houston, TX on March 16-17, 2018. For more details go to bit.ly/godshandcraftedjewels for information and updates.

The following pages are provided for you to use for journaling as you begin your journey of healing. Record what God affirms for you, what thoughts He has toward you in this season and the revelation you gain in the process.

_____
_____
_____
_____
_____
_____
_____
_____
_____
_____
_____
_____
_____
_____
_____
_____

God's Handcrafted Jewel

_____

_____

_____

_____

_____

_____

_____

_____

_____

_____

_____

_____

_____

_____

_____

_____

_____

_____

_____

_____

_____

_____

_____

_____

God's Handcrafted Jewel

God's Handcrafted Jewel

God's Handcrafted Jewel

95

Cathy Jewel Chatman

Cathy Jewel Chatman

God's Handcrafted Jewel

Cathy Jewel Chatman

God's Handcrafted Jewel

Cathy Jewel Chatman

www.ingramcontent.com/pod-product-compliance
Lightning Source LLC
Chambersburg PA
CBHW072204270326
41930CB00011B/2533